DON'T LET THE DR. WAKEFIELD'S

OF THE WORLD CONVINCE YOU TO

ENDANGER YOUR CHILD'S LIFE

Library of congress Control Number: 2021911379

The information in this book is for educational and informational purposes only. Personal medical advice should be discussed with your family physician or pediatrician. The final decision rests entirely with you. The FDA and the CDC usually provide accurate and up-to-date information. Be careful if you feel politics are starting to interfere with sound scientific advice.

I am a strong advocate of life-saving vaccines. Everything in life has risks. Some children and adults have died from vaccines. A lab accident in California caused the accidental release of live polio virus that caused polio and deaths in some Americans. Smallpox has been eliminated by vaccines; the polio vaccine has saved millions of lives and has now almost eliminated polio. Everything in life has risks and benefits. Hopefully this book will help you reach the conclusion that the benefits of vaccines far outweigh the minimal risks.

This book is sold with the understanding that the author is not providing personal medical, legal, or other professional advice. Those decisions should be made through your personal medical education and after consultation with your doctor. Hopefully this book will help with that process.

Thanks to My Great Team

Cover and editing by: Madhobi Rani Ray

Author photograph by:

Website by:

First Edition, 2021

10 9 8 7 6 5 4 3 2 1

This Book Is Dedicated to My Beautiful Wife
Of 52 Years

Amy

DON'T LET THE DR. WAKEFIELD'S
OF THE WORLD CONVINCE YOU TO
ENDANGER YOUR CHILD'S LIFE

Vaccines Can Save You, Your Children, and Grandchildren From Dying

Publisher David L. Grimes MD LLC
www.drdavidlgrimesauthor.com

Introduction

How much is the life of your child or grandchild worth?

This story starts with a milkmaid named Sarah Nelms in 1796. It resulted in the complete elimination of a plague that killed millions of people all over the world. Dr. Jenner developed the first "vaccine" that would go on to save millions of lives around the world. We now have multiple vaccines that prevent over 10,000 deaths every year in the US. We have vaccines that can prevent cancer. Yet, we have parents that have been convinced by quacks that it is safer not to vaccinate their children. They make their children drink the "Jim Jones Kool Aid". This has deadly consequences. This book is being written to help parents and grandparents understand the importance of continuing to use these safe vaccines to save their own lives and their children's lives. It will cover a brief history of vaccine development and the dramatic reduction of diseases and deaths after the use of vaccines became routine. Parents that stopped their children's vaccines, then must live with the guilt if their children catch vaccine preventable diseases and have unnecessary deaths unnecessary deaths.

Decisions have consequences, your child's life may hang in the balance. Many of my parents with new babies or grandchildren have questions about the risks and benefits of vaccines. I have written my first book to make these answers available to everyone concerned about vaccines. This book is based on my 50 years of medical training in obstetrics and public health. Many quacks have convinced parents not to get their child vaccinated, with deadly results. This book reviews the history and safety of vaccines in an easy to understand and read book so parents and grandparents can make an educated decision and not risk the lives of their children.

Understanding research and statistics is complex and often requires college courses and degrees. Common sense, however, can take you a long way. If someone is trying to sell you "miracle hair growing tonic" for several hundred dollars you know to be careful and demand proof. They may say they have three people that will swear that they used the product and "their hair grew like crazy". They may not reveal that the company offered them "all-expense paid vacations around the country" to people that were sure the hair tonic was the solution and were willing to "testify" on TV. This would be different from the company that had independent researchers give 600 partially bald men a six-month trial of medication. Three hundred received the medication and three hundred received a placebo. It was a "randomized, placebo controlled, double blind" experiment. This is the best study that can be done because it avoids bias. Neither the researchers nor the patients knew, until the end of the study, who received the real medicine and who got the placebo. The study showed that there was no difference between the medicine and the placebo in hair growth.

Even with “a money back guarantee”, the miracle tonic is a scam and a waste of your money. People like to convince themselves that something is working even it is not working. Especially, if you wasted a lot of money after your wife told you it was a scam. The other company learned that the product they developed did not work, so they could not sell it.

Unknown to his patients, Dr. Wakefield was being paid secretly by lawyers to collect cases of autism so they could sue the vaccine makers. The lawyers would then take 1/3-2/3 of the millions in lawsuit settlements they would get from suing the vaccine manufactures, for producing a “dangerous” vaccine. Dr. Wakefield collected rare cases of autism. Almost all children were being given the MMR vaccine at this time. He was then able to imply that it was the MMR that caused the autism. He could have easily implied that driving home from the hospital in a car after birth was the cause of autism. The child had autism and the child was driven home in a car.

One plus one always equals two. Parents wanted to believe it was the "bad" vaccine that caused the problem, not something they did or should have done to prevent autism. Noone knows how to prevent autism. Besides, they might make millions of dollars from suing the "bad" vaccine companies that were making millions of dollars in profits. The lawyers convinced them the vaccine companies were only interested in profits and did not care if they caused their child to develop autism. The "bad" vaccine companies had billions of dollars in profits and deserved to pay for their mistakes.

Many researchers pointed out the flaws in Dr. Wakefield's study. They were called "conspirators" on the payroll of the "big bad' vaccine makers. Multiple international studies showed no "cause and effect" between MMR vaccine and autism. Still, parents of children needed someone to blame and continued to prevent their new children from receiving vaccines. Vaccine preventable diseases returned with a vengeance. Children started catching measles again. Children started dying again from a disease that had essentially been eliminated. Brian Deer was an investigative reporter that broke the story and exposed the fraud committed by the lawyers and Dr. Wakefield. His medical article, after review, was repealed and declared "utterly false". Dr. Wakefield lost his UK medical license. He still travels around the world spreading his lies. Some parents, even those highly educated, still place their children at risk by preventing them from getting vaccines.

In 2014 there was a measles epidemic in the Philippines. Two Amish men were returning from the Philippines after doing typhoon relief work. Unknown to them, they were infected with the measles just before leaving to return to Ohio. The Amish typically do not get vaccines even though it is not specifically forbidden by their religion. Typical vaccine rates among the Amish were only 10%. The rate of other Ohio residents was 90%. The epidemic was limited to the Amish community.

Ten thousand Amish were immediately vaccinated, and social gatherings limited until the epidemic resolved. Luckily, there were no deaths. That year the Philippines had over 21,000 cases of the measles and 110 associated measles deaths. Prior to the MMR vaccine there were 500,000 cases of the measles every year in the US and one child died for every 1,000 cases of the measles. Ninety-seven percent (97%) of measles are from unvaccinated foreigners or unvaccinated Americans returning from countries with active measles cases.

Measles epidemics are rare in the US because of the high vaccine rates (90%). This provides "herd immunity". If vaccine rates drop then measles and the associated deaths will return. Most intelligent people do not want to return to the days when over 10,000 children died every year from, what are now, vaccine preventable diseases (VPD). Vaccines are one of the leading causes that one out of ten children no longer die before reaching their first birthday.

We do not have a 'magic single bullet'. Multiple diseases like whooping cough, polio, measles, and others were responsible for the over 10,000 yearly deaths in the US. They each required different vaccines for prevention. That is why so many vaccines are necessary. Some parents say that is "too many" for a baby or young child. Unfortunately, babies or young children sometimes die from these diseases. The only way to get immunity is from a safe vaccine or not die when you get the disease. The "foreign vaccine" injected into your body is safer than the "foreign disease" causing a childhood disease and rarely death. The statistics show a 99% decrease in disease cases and deaths once vaccines became widely used.

Chapter 1

What is the life of your child or grand-child worth?
Choices Have Consequences

The reasons Americans west of the Mississippi do not speak Japanese and those east of the Mississippi do not speak German is because our grandparents and great-grandparents chose not to surrender to pre-war Japan and Nazi Germany. They were willing to resist those ideas with their money and their lives. Some Americans supported Nazi Germany and some also supported Japan. Luckily, most Americans awoke to the danger of flawed socialist and dictator thinking and supported freedom instead. We now have the freedom to make choices for ourselves and our children when it comes to vaccines. If Japan and Nazi Germany had won the war, we would not have the luxury of these choices. The government would make those choices for us. So how do you decide whether to vaccinate or not vaccinate your child? Both sides seem to make logical and scientific appearing recommendations for and against vaccinations. I will try in this book to convince you that it is critically important to have you and your children vaccinated. Many other choices are important. Who should you vote for? Who should control what your children are being taught in school? Should parents have the right to send their children to the school of their choice, including government financial support? Who should oversee your children's and grandchildren's education, you or the teacher's unions? How important is it to teach your children and teenagers about money management and economics in school? Much to our harm, economics and money management has never been taught in our K-12 schools? This book will only focus on the importance, risks, and benefits of vaccines.

What Happens If We Stop Giving Vaccines?

Vaccine choices have consequences. Vaccines may not be the only way to protect your child's life, but they are way ahead of whatever is in second place. Before vaccines were available, diseases like smallpox, whooping cough, polio, measles, haemophilus influenzae and German Measles (rubella) caused widespread disease and thousands of deaths every year in the US. Vaccines have caused dramatic declines and elimination of some of these diseases and their associated deaths. In the early nineteen hundred's (1900's) one (1) out of every ten children born in the United States died before their first birthday. Nearly everyone got the measles and hundreds of children died each year because of the measles. Most of today's new doctors have never even seen a case of the measles. Vaccines now prevent 2 to 3 million deaths in the world every year.

In 1964 to 1965 the US saw an epidemic of

German Measles. Twelve and 1/2 million (12,500,0000) cases occurred and killed over two thousand (2,000) babies. It also caused 11,000 miscarriages. Since 2012 only 15 cases of German Measles have been reported and most of these were brought in from outside the country. Diphtheria caused almost 21,000 cases each year in the United States with almost one in every ten children dying from this disease. Polio caused 36,000 cases a year, again with almost one out of every ten children dying from this disease. Once we developed successful vaccines, we have seen almost total elimination of these diseases and deaths.

Most diseases are spread from one non-immune or non-vaccinated person to another. A vaccinated person cannot catch or spread these diseases. People that had the disease and recovered are also immune, but they could have been seriously injured or died from the disease. Vaccines make you immune without making you sick or killing you. Over 90% of vaccine-preventable diseases are now brought into our country from foreign travelers and legal and illegal aliens that have the disease. They have not been required to have proof of vaccines or been required to obtain vaccines before being allowed into our country. We only need to look at the southern US border today to see the problems. Because America is the home of the free, we should not make vaccines mandatory. However, we should require all foreign nationals traveling to or migrating to our country to have these vaccines. This is for our protection as well as theirs. We should do everything to educate native-born Americans about the importance and safety of vaccines. When we are in epidemics, almost everyone wants the vaccine to keep from dying or developing serious complications. When the country has been safe for years, because of these vaccines, we seem to think that they are optional. It is like the joke of the beatnik standing on the corner of Hollywood and Vine and snapping his fingers. A policeman approached and asked him "What are you doing?" He replies, "I am keeping the elephants away." The policeman replies but there are no elephants here. The beatnik replies, "See it's working". Just because thousands of children and adults are not dying from these vaccine-preventable diseases every year, does not mean that we need to stop giving the vaccines. It is only when the diseases have been eliminated that we can stop these vaccines.

In Japan in 1970 about 80% of children were getting a whooping cough vaccine and only 393 cases were seen, with no deaths. Since few cases were seen parents began questioning if the vaccine was even necessary. Vaccine rates dropped dramatically to only 10%. In 1979 13,000 Japanese got whooping cough and 41 (mostly babies) died. Vaccination rates went back up and the epidemic and deaths disappeared. Parents had to live with the guilt that they had caused their babies death by not getting themselves and their children vaccinated. Getting yourself and your children vaccinated keeps not only you and your children safe, but future generations as well.

Everyone has heard of the swine and bird flu. Smallpox was a disease only found in humans and was eliminated with the smallpox vaccine. We will never be able to eliminate the flu. Pigs and birds carry the same flu virus as humans and will always keep giving it back to us because they carry the same virus. However, if we eliminate smallpox (which has been done) and polio (which has almost been done) then we can stop those vaccines because humans are the only ones that can carry those diseases. By keeping up our defenses with vaccines, we are currently preventing 2 to 3 million deaths worldwide every year. Still more than 1.5 million people die every year from diseases that could have been prevented with vaccines.

We now have vaccines that can prevent 17 different diseases. Most children recover from measles, mumps, and chickenpox. However, despite great scientific discoveries and new treatments, many still died unnecessarily without the vaccine. Sick children may require parents to miss work and the children to get behind in school. It is estimated that childhood vaccines save over 33,000 lives, prevent 14 million cases of disease, and save billions of dollars in health care costs. In the US 42,000 adults and over 300 children die each year that could have been prevented with available vaccines.

As you might have guessed I am not an anti-vaxxer. I will provide the facts that support my view. If you are strongly opposed to vaccines for your children, you will probably not read this book and be confused or brainwashed with "fake" facts. You may not realize the fact that the reason you did not die from smallpox, polio, flu, measles, whooping cough, and tetanus as a child was because your parents and grandparents made sure you were given the safe and necessary vaccines to prevent these diseases. Can some children live until their 70's without ever having been vaccinated against these deadly diseases? Of course, they can and did, even back in the 1600's, 1700's, 1800's, and 1900's some children did live until their 70s. Many unnecessary deaths occurred that can now be prevented with today's modern and safe vaccines.

Would your odds of being alive today be better with or without vaccines? Even if these diseases did not kill you, would you be less likely or more likely to be in an iron lung (polio), have permanent paralysis (polio), have birth defects (German Measles) and have horrible skin scarring (smallpox)? I hope this book can help you learn and understand the importance of these decisions for you and more importantly for your children. Your parents and grandparents made sure you and your parents were safe. You have the sole responsibility to make sure your children have the best chance of living a safer and longer life. Historically we have good data on the number of children that died or had serious diseases before and after vaccines.

Chapter 2
A Brief History of Vaccines

Sarah Nelms was a milkmaid in 1796 working for a wealthy landowner. Milkmaids commonly develop lesions on their hands and arms. These lesions were caused from cows having cowpox. Many people had observed that milkmaids seldom got or died from the dreaded smallpox epidemics. These epidemics killed an average of 500,000 people each year in Europe and around the world. These epidemics had been going on for centuries. Old Egyptian mummies had evidence of smallpox. In addition to no known treatment or prevention, there was a lifetime of scarring that was associated with surviving this disease. Survivors were immune and unable to catch the disease again during recurrent epidemics. Dr. Edward Jenner was the landowner's doctor and had heard of giving people cowpox or even smallpox to prevent them from dying from smallpox. Giving people smallpox to keep them from dying from smallpox does not seem to make much sense. Cowpox was a mild disease, but smallpox was often fatal. He took fluid from Sarah's hand lesions and placed it in a scratch on the arm of the owner's 8-year-old son. The boy had only a small reaction. Months later he inoculated the boy with smallpox and the boy had only a mild reaction but did not develop smallpox or cowpox. Several months later he again challenged the boy with smallpox and the boy had no reaction at all. He was immune to smallpox without ever having had the disease or the risk of dying.

Dr Jenner then began inoculating adults and children in the area with cowpox. He wrote one of the first medical papers in the world on the benefit of a "vaccine" to prevent smallpox. He did not know that cowpox and smallpox were viruses from the same family of viruses. No one knew that viruses even existed at this time. He did know that cowpox was mild, and smallpox was deadly. He also knew that milkmaids seldom got smallpox even during epidemics. His experiment would never pass today's safety standards and never be allowed. However, when entire towns were being wiped out by these recurring smallpox epidemics many things were being tried to treat or prevent these epidemics. Most were unsuccessful. Dr. Jenner's cowpox vaccine was the first method that consistently reduced the risk of death and disease. It led to the eventual complete elimination of smallpox. There are now no longer any cases of smallpox on earth. Cowpox became the first successful vaccine to prevent a disease. Inoculation with a similar but weaker live virus prevented the deadly smallpox.

The last case of smallpox was in 1977 in Somalia. We still manufacture the smallpox vaccine in case it is ever needed. The US and Russia have the only remaining live cultures of the smallpox virus. Therefore, there is still a small risk that will always exist that terrorists could try to restart the disease with germ warfare. An accidental exposure in a US lab resulted in the death of a lab worker from smallpox in 1978. The last case of wild smallpox in the US was in 1949. The US stopped giving smallpox vaccines in 1972. When 500,000 people each year were dying from smallpox there were very few people against the only known vaccine or treatment that could prevent them and their children from dying or having horrible permanent scarring. Cowpox was the first successful vaccine and has now resulted in the total elimination of the dreaded disease of smallpox from our world.

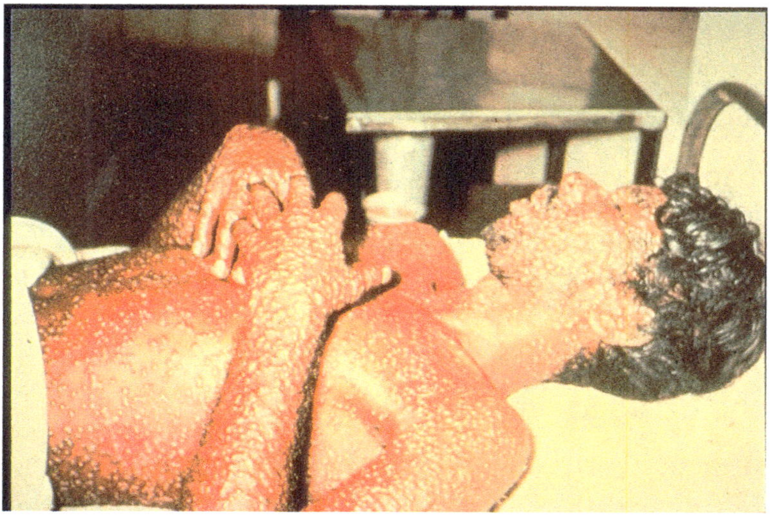

Adult with smallpox from CDC files

Dr. Louis Pasteur in the late eighteen hundreds went on to develop vaccines against chicken cholera and rabies. Even more amazing was the fact that germs like bacteria and viruses were still unknown because they were too small to see, and no microscopes were available at this time.

The Polio Vaccine

We have now also almost eliminated polio. In 1952 America had its worst polio outbreak. There were 58,000 cases and 3,000 deaths. There were 21,000 cases of paralysis with entire hospital wards of children and adults in the dreaded "iron lungs" because they were unable to breathe on their own. I remember getting the "shot" in second grade. Kids (and a lot of adults) do not like needles or shots. My boyhood friend was not as lucky and was in an iron lung, and after recovery, a wheelchair for the rest of his life. The few minutes of pain from the shot was well worth not being in an iron lung and a wheelchair for the rest of my life or dying. President Roosevelt was also a victim of polio and required a wheelchair. I remember roller skating through downtown Tampa, Florida in sixth grade collecting money in cans for the "March of Dimes" and polio research. Polio is gone from the western hemisphere. The March of Dimes is still collecting money. Research is now to prevent birth defects since polio has been defeated.

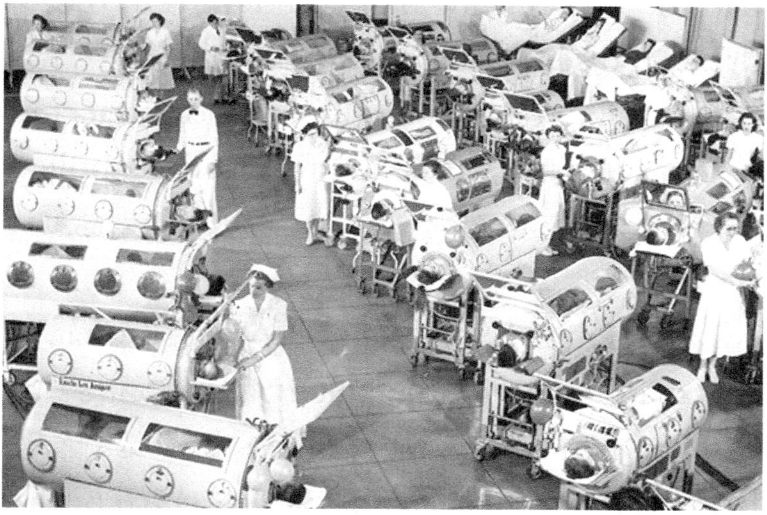

Lives Lost from Vaccines

Dr. Jonas Salk developed and released the first polio vaccine on February 23,1954. At this time, the only fear of vaccines was that there might not be enough vaccines for all parents and their children. Doctor Salk made his vaccine by growing the virus in monkey kidneys. He then killed the whole virus in a formaldehyde solution before it was injected into humans. He first tested the vaccine on himself, his wife, and his children. Thus, we had the first vaccine that could prevent the dreaded disease called polio. In 1962 Dr. Albert Sabin developed the oral polio vaccine. It was a live but weakened form of the polio virus.

An accident in 1955 in a California lab that was manufacturing the killed Salk vaccine resulted in a batch that still had the live virus being accidentally given to people. Five people died and 51 were paralyzed. This resulted in many people being against vaccines. If the polio vaccine had been stopped, instead of the problem corrected, many more people would have died or been paralyzed from this horrible disease. Just because people die in car accidents does not mean that all cars need to be parked and never driven again. Instead, we have worked to develop safer cars with seat belts and airbags. We make drivers safer by not allowing drinking or using cell phones while driving. By the same logic we continue working to improve and make all vaccines safer and more effective. Newer and safer vaccines are being developed every day.

Children liked the oral polio vaccine better because it was on a sugar cube instead of the dreaded shot. The oral polio vaccine gave better immunity because it was a live but weakened virus that reproduced in your body like a natural infection, but it still gave good immunity without disease. A live weakened infection gives a stronger immune response because the strong virus may kill or injure you. A killed vaccine cannot multiply in your body, therefore creating a weaker immune response, but still adequate in most cases. A vaccine is designed to give you immunity to the disease without making you sick. The main drawback to the oral polio virus was that in rare cases it could spontaneously revert to the original deadly virus (1-5 cases in a million vaccines) and give you polio. This could probably have been prevented by giving them the killed shot first and then following up with the stronger oral vaccine. I received the shot (Salk vaccine) in second grade while going to school in Kentucky. When we moved back to Florida, I received the sugar cube (Sabin vaccine). The oral polio vaccine is no longer available in the US because the shot is safer. "Double vaccine" is probably not necessary because we have now almost eliminated polio from the world. Poor countries may be unable to afford "double" vaccines. The oral vaccine was also cheaper and easier to transport and administer. It is easier and cheaper for poor countries to give a child a sugar cube than hiring nurses and doctors to give shots.

The last wild case of polio originating in the US was in 1979. The last case brought into the US by foreign travelers was in 1993. Hopefully, polio will become the second disease totally eliminated from our world and the polio vaccine will no longer be needed. It is now more important than ever that foreigners crossing our borders legally or illegally be screened for multiple diseases, have records of vaccinations, or be vaccinated if uncertain before exposure to the people in our country.

Lives Saved

Immunizations currently prevent 2 to 3 million deaths every year. In early 1900, one out of every ten children born in the United States died before their first birthday. More than 1.5 million people worldwide die each year from vaccine-preventable diseases. Either the vaccine was not available, or parents refused it for themselves and their children. Most childhood deaths in the United States are not due to lack of availability of the vaccine, but due to parents who have 'drank the Kool-Aid' of Dr. Wakefield. The CDC has estimated that one child dies worldwide every 20 seconds from a vaccine-preventable disease. Even in wealthy countries with available vaccines, like the US and Japan, parents have become complacent and unnecessary deaths have resulted from diseases such as whooping cough and diphtheria. California recently had several babies die from whooping cough, a totally preventable death with the whooping cough vaccine. We now vaccinate all pregnant women during pregnancy for whooping cough. We also recommend that dad, grandparents, and anyone that is going to be around the baby during the first few months of life be given the Tdap (tetanus, diphtheria and acellular pertussis) vaccine booster while mom is still pregnant. Acellular pertussis is another name for whooping cough. This will protect the baby after birth until it is old enough to be given the DTap vaccine and develop its own immunity.

The new covid-19 vaccines have again raised questions of safety. Do they work? Were they developed "too fast"? Despite their rapid development, they appear to be very effective and very safe. The rapid but safe development of these vaccines has saved thousands of lives and prevented much suffering. Many politicians recommended taking years to develop these vaccines. When millions of people are dying from an epidemic, you do not wait 3 years to develop the "safest" vaccine. President Trump was able to work with the pharmaceutical companies to develop a rapid but safe vaccine in record time that saved millions of lives.

The Pfizer vaccine was compared to a placebo shot in over 40,000 people. One hundred and seventy (170) people developed covid-19. One hundred and sixty two (162) of these were in the placebo group and only eight were(8) in the vaccine group. Four (4) deaths occurred in the placebo group and only 2 in the vaccine group. If 2 people die 6 months after going to a stock car race we do not blame going to the race for their deaths. The scientific review committee of doctors and scientists did not find any correlation between the vaccine and the expected deaths. This showed an effectiveness of over 95% in preventing covid, admission to ICU, and death from covid. If you are over 70 and choose not to get the covid vaccine that is your right as an American. But why would you want to die from a disease that could be prevented with a safe and effective vaccine? If you have had the vaccine or the disease you are no longer at risk for catching the disease again or giving it to anyone else. Masks are not necessary. If you are young and choose not to get the vaccine you may get sick but most likely will not die. The same is true of the flu shot. If you are young, you are unlikely to die from the flu but why be miserable for a week when it could be prevented with the vaccine. Diseases that can kill you or make you seriously ill, but can be prevented with vaccines deserve your thought and attention.

The Maderna vaccine was given to over 28,000 people. There were 185 cases in the placebo group and only 11 cases of covid in the vaccine group. This effectiveness has been shown to be much better than the flu vaccine. We are uncertain at this time if annual booster shots will be necessary, and we'll probably have to recommend annual boosters until we have enough time to find out if it is really necessary.

When considering the effectiveness and safety of vaccines it is important to look at the historical data. The table below looks at US cases and deaths, both pre and post vaccine and the percent reduction in deaths with the development and utilization of vaccines. Why would any parent want to risk their child dying when it could easily be prevented with a proven safe vaccine?

Table-1: US Yearly Cases And Deaths (Averages from CDC)

	Pre Vaccine Cases	Pre Vaccine Deaths	Post Vaccine Cases	Post Vaccine Deaths	% Deaths decreased
Disease					
Smallpox	29,000	337 (500,000 worldwide)	0	0	100%
Polio (acute)	20,000	1,400	0	0	100%
Polio (paralytic)	16,000	2,000	0	0	100%
Diphtheria	21,000	2,000	0	0	100%
Measles	530,000	440	55	0	100%
Mumps	162,000	39	6,500	0	100%
Whooping Cough	200,000	4,000	15,000	27	99%
German Measles	48,000	17	11	0	100%
Tetanus	580	472	41	4	99%
Totals	**1,026,580**	**10,705**	**21,607**	**31**	**99%**

The Dr. Wakefield Disaster

The main reason parents in wealthy countries prevent their children and themselves from getting life-saving vaccines is lack of scientific understanding and being scammed by quacks. In February 1998 a British doctor by the name of Dr. Andrew Wakefield published a medical paper that "supposedly" showed that the MMR (measles, mumps, and rubella) vaccine caused inflammation in the bowel and autism in children. That was very scary to parents and caused many of them to stop vaccinating their children. Dr. Wakefield was exposed 6 years later as a fraud by a newspaper reporter named Brian Deer. His investigation found that Dr. Wakefield had been paid by lawyers to find cases in order to sue the vaccine companies, not do valid scientific research. He falsified the information in his research paper to make it look like a legitimate research paper. Multiple studies in many countries have subsequently been done and proven that there is absolutely no connection between the MMR vaccine and autism. But the damage had already been done. Many parents were convinced (and some still believe) that the MMR vaccine might cause autism in their children and prevented their children from getting these life-saving vaccines.

The fraudulent article was removed and declared "utterly false". Dr. Wakefield was found guilty of serious medical research misconduct in 2010 and barred from practicing medicine in the UK. Unfortunately, because of Dr. Wakefield, the lack of children getting the MMR during this time resulted in deaths and serious permanent injuries to unvaccinated children. Dr. Wakefield was also found to have filed a patent for a "safer" vaccine that would have made him millions of dollars if he could have falsely convinced doctors and parents that the MMR was not safe. He then founded a "treatment center" for children with autism in Texas in 2004 but resigned in 2010 after the UK investigation resulted in the loss of his UK medical license. His wife of 32 years divorced him after he left her for supermodel Elle Macpherson. Who says, "scams don't pay (very well)"? How many deaths and serious permanent injuries can be attributed to the "king of the anti- vaxxers"? How many people still listen to this discredited quack? Do not let Dr. Wakefield convince you not to vaccinate your children and make them drink the "Jim Jones Kool-Aid". Do not be responsible for your child dying from a vaccine-preventable disease.

Suspected deaths after vaccines are always reviewed and medical records and autopsy reports checked for, if available. Most are found to be unrelated (motor vehicle accidents or other causes) or have other more likely causes rather than the vaccine. Sudden infant death syndrome (SIDS) peaked in 1992 to 1993. Most were caused by babies being put to sleep on their tummies. With the "Back to Sleep" campaign we saw dramatic decreases in deaths, despite increasing numbers of vaccines. There were fewer infant deaths. If vaccines were the cause, we would have expected to see it increase in the number of infant deaths with more vaccines being given. SIDS and childhood vaccines occur in the same age groups. "Vaccine-associated deaths" also had twice as many low-birth-weight babies. Low birth-weight babies have a higher risk of death for up to two years old. Multiple scientific reviews of infant death reports have found no consistent pattern of a causal relationship between vaccinations and death. A study in 2013 of 13 million vaccinated children, 1 to 2 months after vaccination, showed no difference in death rates when compared to the US general population. The causes of death in both groups were essentially the same. All these studies provided convincing evidence that vaccines were associated with a decrease in death and disease rather than an increase. A few deaths have resulted as a direct result from vaccines (allergic reactions and children with congenital immune deficiencies). Many more lives are saved than lost from vaccines. All this information can be confirmed at the CDC vaccine website and on the internet. Please do your own independent research.

Chapter 3

The First Vaccines To Prevent Cancer

Hepatitis A, B, and C

In 1981 the hepatitis B (HepB) vaccine became the first vaccine that could prevent cancer. Chronic Hepatitis B was the leading cause of liver cancer. If a pregnant patient has hepatitis B (chronic or acute), the baby most likely would develop chronic Hepatitis B from going through the birth canal. If the newborn baby gets hepatitis B from the mother at birth, it has a high chance of being a chronic lifetime carrier of hepatitis B. We think the newborn's immune system is fooled into thinking that Hepatitis B is a part of the baby's body and therefore does not attack the virus. The virus then continues to grow throughout the life of the individual. It attacks the liver and eventually that person can develop liver cancer. Sixty percent (60%) of liver cancers were due to cases of chronic hepatitis B. Fifteen (15%) to twenty-five (25%) percent of infants with chronic hepatitis B will die prematurely from cirrhosis, liver failure, or liver cancer.

In 1991, the hepatitis B vaccine was recommended for all infants born in the US. All pregnant women were tested for acute and chronic Hepatitis B. Pregnant women with hepatitis B were treated and the newborn was given extra protection called Hepatitis B immune globulin or HBIG. The first of three Hepatitis B vaccines was also given to the newborn at birth. This kept most infants from becoming chronic Hepatitis B carriers and dying from liver disease and liver cancer. The original vaccine was made by inactivating Hepatitis B from Hepatitis B carriers with heat and formaldehyde which killed the virus. The newest Hepatitis B is a genetically engineered DNA recombinant vaccine and does not contain any blood products. It is impossible to get Hepatitis B from the newest vaccine. More evidence that we continue to make vaccines safer.

Hepatitis B has declined 90% since the introduction of the vaccine and HBIG. In 1982 there were 9 .6 cases for every hundred thousand people (9.6/100,000). In 2018 this declined to only one (1/100,000) case for every hundred thousand people. This represents a decline of almost 90% of the cases. Most cases of hepatitis B in the US now come from foreign immigrants. Testing of immigrants is recommended but not enforced. Immigrants waiting to migrate to the US legally should be required to provide evidence of vaccinations or be vaccinated while they are waiting to get legal permission to migrate to the US. We should require our government to vaccinate all illegal immigrants crossing our southern border before being released into the United States.
Seventy-five percent (75%) of newborns in the US now received their first dose of Hepatitis B at birth. Ninety percent (90%) have been

fully vaccinated by age 2. Intravenous drug users from needle sharing are increasing the rates of hepatitis B. Because of the decrease in cases of hepatitis B from the vaccine, hepatitis C (Hep C) now has become the leading cause of liver cancer. There has not been a dramatic increase in cases of hepatitis C. Because of the successful hepatitis B vaccine, we have seen a dramatic decrease in cases of hepatitis B. This now leaves hepatitis C as the leading cause of liver cancer.

Unlike hepatitis A and hepatitis B, hepatitis C does not yet have a vaccine. However, we can now cure hepatitis C. Seventy-five percent (75%) of hepatitis C carriers were born between 1945 and 1965 (i.e., baby boomers). Hepatitis C is not usually spread like hepatitis B by sex. Blood and needle sharing appear to be the greatest risk for contracting hepatitis C. Children born to mothers with hepatitis C are also at high risk of developing this disease during birth. Hepatitis C can now easily be cured with a single pill taken daily for two to three months even though no vaccine is yet available. Fifty percent (50%) of all US liver cancer cases are now caused by hepatitis C because Hep B is on the way to being eliminated. If you were born between 1945 and 1965, went to Woodstock, or used IV drugs please get tested. Hepatitis C is often asymptomatic (you do not feel sick).

If you have never had vaccines for Hepatitis A and B you can safely receive them before or even during pregnancy. Any killed vaccine is safer than having the disease during pregnancy. The live vaccines should be given before or after pregnancy. Most will probably not harm the baby if you accidentally get pregnant in less than a month after the vaccine. Live attenuated vaccines include MMR, the flu nasal vaccine, the oral polio vaccine, the BCG (TB) vaccine and varicella (Chickenpox or shingles).

Cervical Cancer

Cervical cancer has always been a killer of young women. With the invention of the pap smear we were able to detect and treat dysplasia. Dysplasia is the pre-malignant change on the cervix that often occurs years before it progresses into cancer. Dysplasia is easy to cure, cervical cancer is not easy to cure Even with Pap smear screening available we still see 11,000 cases of cervical cancer each year and 4,000 deaths in the US because of women not getting their regular pap smears. By easily treating and eliminating dysplasia we were able to prevent progression to cervical cancer.

Cervical cancer and dysplasia are caused by multiple types of the human papilloma virus (HPV). Type 16 and 18 are responsible for 70% of all cervical cancers worldwide. The newest HPV vaccine (Gardasil 9) can prevent 90% of all cervical and penile cancers. It also prevents condylomas which are genital warts that are caused by type 6 and 11 HPV. The

HPV vaccine became the second vaccine that could prevent cancer. HPV vaccines became available in 2006. HPV is a sexually transmitted virus. The vaccine only works if given before exposure to the virus. The HPV vaccine is now recommended for all children between the ages of 9 and 13. Regular pap smears are still recommended because the vaccine only prevents 90% of cervical cancer cases. Poor countries may not be able to afford regular pap smears for their female population. The HPV vaccine may be the only cost-effective alternative. The Pap smear can still catch the 10% of cases missed by the vaccine or in the unvaccinated children.

Chapter 4

Childhood Vaccines

Discuss vaccine recommendations with your pediatrician or family doctor. Keep in mind the pre and post vaccine table showing cases and deaths that could be prevented with vaccines. Believe it or not, the baby can be given immunity from disease even before it is born. Mom's immunity from disease or vaccines is passively transferred across the placenta to the baby. This passive immunity- will usually slowly disappear and is gone by 1 year of age. Any disease that mom is immune to, the baby will also be immune to, at least for a short time after birth. Before the baby loses its passive immunity from mom, the baby needs to be vaccinated to be able to produce its own antibodies (active immunity) and protection from these diseases.

Whooping Cough (acellular pertussis)

Most babies dying from whooping cough are younger than 2 months old. Because of this we now give all pregnant women between the 7th and 8th month of pregnancy the Tdap vaccine that contains the vaccine for whooing cough. The Tdap vaccine is 3 vaccines in one. It contains a vaccine for tetanus, diphtheria and acellular pertussis (whooping cough). Vaccines have germs or pieces of germs called antigens that have been killed or weakened so that they are unable to cause disease. These trigger our body to make proteins called antibodies that attack and kill these germs. The baby's immune system also "remembers" the germs for years or a lifetime and can then attack and kill the germs before they have a chance to cause a new case of the disease. Once a child has had the measles or the measles vaccine, they usually cannot ever get the measles again.

The passive antibody transfer from mom

saves the life of the newborn baby that would not have time to make its own antibodies or be immunized. Dad and grandparents or anyone around the newborn baby also need to be sure they have had a recent Tdap vaccine while mom is still pregnant so they will not be able to give the baby whooping cough, even if they have no symptoms. This is saving many babies' lives. The baby then gets its whooping cough vaccine (DTap) at two months of age. Within a few weeks after the vaccine the baby can develop its own immune response and fight off this disease. We recommend the Tdap vaccine every 10 years for all individuals over 10 years of age. DTap and Tdap are often confused. They have the same ingredients but different strengths. DTaP is stronger and is used for initial immunization of children 6 weeks to 7 years old. Tdap is weaker and used as a booster shot for anyone over 10 years of age. The booster shots do not need to be as strong. Both shots prevent the same diseases (diphtheria, tetanus, and whooping cough).

US Disease	Pre-Vaccine Cases	Pre-Vaccine Deaths	Post Vaccine Cases	Post Vaccine Deaths	% Deaths decreased
Whooping Cough	200,000	4,000	15,000	27	99%

Polio

Prior to the invention of the polio vaccine there were almost 40,000 cases in the US each year and about 3,500 deaths each year. The days of iron lungs, paralysis and deaths from this disease were eliminated mainly because our grandparents and parents made sure we received the polio vaccine. Hopefully, the disease will soon be only of historical significance and the disease will become the second one eliminated from this world. Then the polio vaccine will no longer be necessary.

US Disease	Pre-Vaccine Cases	Pre-Vaccine Deaths	Post Vaccine Cases	Post Vaccine Deaths	% Deaths decreased
Polio (acute)	20,000	1,400	0	0	100%
Polio (paralytic)	16,000	2,000	0	0	100%

Diphtheria

Before the vaccine there were 21,000 cases and 2,000 deaths in the US every year from diphtheria. Since the vaccine we no longer have any recorded cases or deaths from this disease. This represents a 100% decrease since the invention of the diphtheria vaccine. Without the continued use of the vaccine, it will come back with a vengeance.

US Disease	Pre-Vaccine Cases	Pre-Vaccine Deaths	Post Vaccine Cases	Post Vaccine Deaths	% Deaths decreased
Diphtheria	21,000	2,000	0	0	100%

Flu Shot

Mom and every family member also need the flu shot during pregnancy and yearly. This protects not only mom but the baby as well. In 2009 the swine flu (H1N1) had one of the highest mortality rates in pregnant women when compared to other groups. If mom dies early in pregnancy then so does the baby.The flu virus rapidly changes every year (in humans, birds,and pigs). Because of this, scientists are required to develop a new flu shot on a yearly basis. The nasal flu vaccine is a live attenuated virus so theoretically should not be used during pregnancy. The flu shot is a killed flu virus and has been proven safe for pregnant patients. During the 2017 to the 2018 flu season the CDC estimated that with only a 40% vaccination rate the US still prevented 6.2 million cases of the flu and 5,700 deaths. With a 100% vaccination rate we could have prevented over 15 million cases and almost 15,000 deaths in adults and chil- dren.

Measles

Measles is one of the most infectious diseases known to man. Before the vaccine we saw over 500,000 cases in the US every year. This resulted in 440 children dying every year from a "simple childhood disease". Many parents do not believe that a "simple childhood disease" could be responsible for killing their child. Over 10,000 children died every year in the US prior to vaccines becoming available. By that same token, we can now prevent 10,000 of our precious children each year from dying with the use of all available childhood vaccines. Do not let Dr. Wakefield convince you to let your child die by not getting these safe vaccines. Measles and German Measles are caused by different viruses and cause different diseases.

US Disease	Pre-Vaccine Cases	Pre-Vaccine Deaths	Post Vaccine Cases	Post Vaccine Deaths	% Deaths decreased
Measles	530,000	440	55	0	100%

German Measles (Rubella)

German Measles (rubella) in early pregnancy can cause serious birth defects and miscarriages. Congenital rubella syndrome can cause the baby to be born blind, have hearing loss, heart defects, mental retardation and a small head(microcephaly). Since the vaccine is a weakened, but live virus, we recommend not giving it during pregnancy. This is because of theoretical safety factors for the baby. However, women that accidentally got pregnant sooner than one month after the MMR (measles, mumps, and rubella) vaccine have not seen these birth defects. To be safe we still recommend getting the vaccine before pregnancy or after pregnancy. Most young pregnant women received the vaccine as a child and are protected. If your parents believed Dr. Wakefield and you never received the MMR or chickenpox vaccine, please get the MMR and chickenpox vaccine at least one month before stopping your birth control to prevent your child from having these horrible birth defects and you from dying.

US Disease	Pre-Vaccine Cases	Pre-Vaccine Deaths	Post Vaccine Cases	Post Vaccine Deaths	% Deaths decreased
German Measles	48,000	17	11	0	100%

Mumps

I remember the swollen jaws as a child. I did not feel sick but enjoyed getting to stay home from school and watch cartoons. Luckily, I did not get the complication of swollen testicles and possible sterilization that some friends did suffer. Prior to the vaccine becoming available, over a hundred and fifty thousand cases (162,000) occurred every year in the US and about 40 deaths. Since that vaccine has become available, we are only seeing 6,500 cases each year and no deaths.

US Disease	Pre-Vaccine Cases	Pre-Vaccine Deaths	Post Vaccine Cases	Post Vaccine Deaths	% Deaths decreased
Mumps	162,000	39	6,500	0	100%

Hib (Haemophilus influenzae type b)

Hib can cause severe illness and meningitis in children less than 5. Prior to the Hib vaccines we saw 20,000 cases each year and 1,000 deaths. The Hib vaccine can be combined into one shot with diphtheria, tetanus, pertussis (whooping cough), polio, and hepatitis B. The series requires 3 or 4 shots for Hib. Prior to the Hib vaccine, it was the leading cause of bacterial meningitis (infection of the lining of the brain and spine) in children. Before the vaccine was available, Hib was responsible for 95% of all H. influenza infections. The Hib vaccine has been responsible for a 99% decrease in cases and deaths from Hib.

US Disease	Pre-Vaccine Cases	Pre-Vaccine Deaths	Post Vaccine Cases	Post Vaccine Deaths	% Deaths decreased
Hib	20,000	1,000	50		>99%

Rotavirus (RV)

Rotavirus is given as oral drops (2-3 doses) to prevent severe diarrhea and vomiting in babies. Severe diarrhea and vomiting can result in death.

Pneumococcal conjugate vaccine (PCV13)

PCV13 prevents some types of strep infections. These infections can cause pneumonia, meningitis, and other serious infections. Four doses at 2,4,6, and 12 months are needed. The vaccine protects against 13 strains of pneumococcus. Unvaccinated adults usually only need a single lifetime dose.

CDC Childhood Recommended Vaccine Schedule

These are now all preventable diseases and deaths. Parents need to remain vigilant because if they let down their guard and stop vaccinating their children these diseases will return with a vengeance. Japan learned this lesson the hard way. When parents became complacent about vaccines, childhood diseases and deaths returned. I feel sad for the parents that had a child that died from a disease that could have been prevented with a simple and safe vaccine.
Below is the current CDC recommended schedule for childhood vaccinations. Please visit their website.

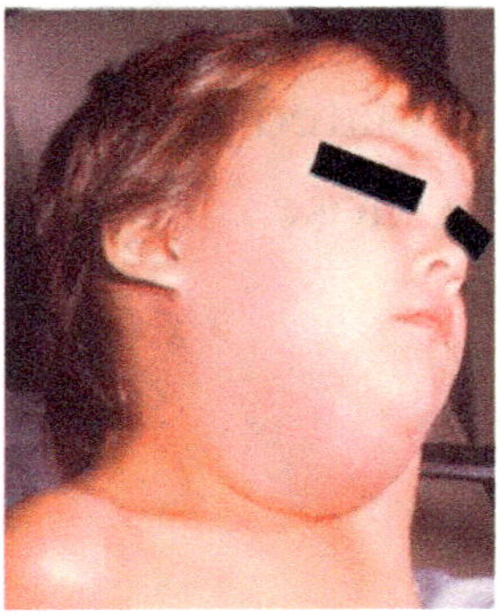

CDC photo of child with mumps

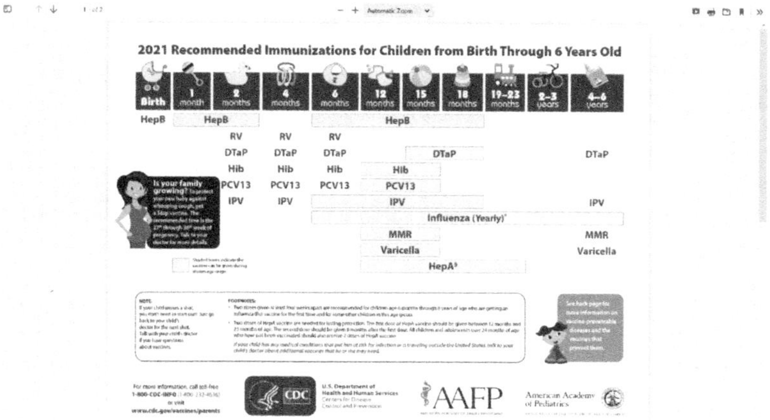
2021 Recommended Immunizations for Children from Birth Through 6 Years Old
Birth
1 month
2 months
4 months
6 months
12 months
15 months
18 months
19–23 months
2–3 years
4–6 years
HepB
HepB
HepB
RV
RV
RV
DTaP
DTaP
DTaP
DTaP
DTaP
Hib
Hib
Hib
Hib
PCV13
PCV13
PCV13
PCV13
IPV
IPV
IPV
IPV
Influenza (Yearly)
MMR
MMR
Varicella
Varicella
HepA
Is your family growing?
CDC
AAFP
American Academy of Pediatrics
www.cdc.gov/vaccines/parents

The End

Thanks

• For taking the time to read my book
• If you have any questions, feel free to contact me through my website and sign up for my free monthly newsletter
• www.DrDavidLGrimesAuthor.com
• As a new author I would greatly appreciate a brief review of this book on Amazon or your purchase site if you have time
• Let me know which book you prefer I write next
• I wish to thank all of the doctors and scientists that have made these great discoveries possible and for all of the lives they have saved
• I even thank Dr. Salk for the shot I received in second grade that I did not like then, I still liked Dr. Sabin's sugar cube better
• I am glad I did not wind-up dead, paralyzed, or in an iron lung and thank them both very much
• If you liked this book, please consider sending a copy as a gift to your children, grandchildren, and loved ones---You may save a life
• I wish to thank all of the great doctors at Wilford Hall (USAF); Col. Alvin "Bud" Brekken, Col. Bob Harris, Col. Fred Massey, Col. Don Gambrell, Col. John Hauth, Lt. Col George Hilliard, and my favorite "intern" Col. Gary Hankins. They made me a better doctor than I ever thought I could be.

Acknowledgement Page

- This book was not written as a medical text, it has no footnotes or references
- The CDC has an excellent website for understanding vaccines, their risks and benefits (they messed up on facemasks and locking kids out of school but did a great job on vaccines)
- Google Vaccine Preventable Diseases (VPD)

- For detailed information on Dr. Wakefield (Ctrl + click) below:

The Doctor Who Fooled the World: Science, Deception, and the War on Vaccines

by Brian Deer, Dennis Kleinman, et al.
- Please always discuss vaccines with your family doctor or pediatrician (after you read my book), so they can help convince you of the importance vaccines play in saving your and your child's life

Free Monthly Newsletter Sign Up

If you would like a free monthly newsletter, coming publications with sample chapters, please go to my website:

www.drdavidlgrimesauthor.com

Coming Publications

1. How to Prevent Dying from Cancer
2. Osteoporosis, Or Who Gets All the Breaks
3. Preventing Cardiovascular Disease (CVD)
4. Preventing Unplanned Pregnancies
5. How Planned Pregnancies Can Keep Your Baby Healthy
6. Women and Their Hormones
7. Why Your Teens Need Competent Sex Education
8. Why Are We All Not Having Great Sex
9. Why Diabetes Is Affecting 50% of Our Population, And How You Can Prevent Dying from It

About The Author

Dr. Grimes grew up in Tampa, FL and graduated from King High School in Temple Terrace, FL (suburb of Tampa). He graduated from the Univ. of KY with a BS in Medical Technology. He graduated from the Univ. of KY College of Medicine with a MD degree. He graduated from the Univ. of KY College of Public Health with a MPH degree. Needless to say UK Wildcat Blue is his favorite color. He is a Lifetime Fellow of ACOG.

He served in the USAF for 11 years. He completed his OB/GYN residency at Wilford Hall USAF at Lackland AFB in San Antonio, TX. He was on the hospital staff at Clark AFB in the Philippines at the end of the Vietnam War. He returned to a teaching position at Wilford Hall until going into private practice in Greenville, KY and Paducah, KY, his wife's hometown. He became Medical Director of Family Health for the Arkansas Department of Health and now runs a consulting medical practice and lives with his wife in Hot Springs Village, AR.

Dr. Grimes has three children and three grandchildren.

Made in the USA
Monee, IL
03 November 2026

67380051R00046